SHORTS TEQNIQUES OF KUNG FU

By Gulzar Ahmad

Contents

Introduction.

Straight Punch (Jik Chong Chui): A direct punch executed with the lead hand, focusing on speed andaccuracy.
Palm Strike (Zhang Chui): A strike delivered with an open hand, using the palm as the striking surface.
Front Kick (Chun Tui): A powerful kick executed by raising the knee and extending the leg straight forward.
Side Kick (Yao Tui): A kick delivered by extending the leg out to the side while maintainingbalance.
Roundhouse Kick (Waai Tui): A circular kick where the leg is swung around in a horizontal arc to strike the opponent.
Elbow Strike (Zhou Chui): A close-range strike using the elbow, typically directed at the opponent's vital areas.
Knee Strike (Tui Chui): A strike using the knee, performed by raising the knee and driving it into thetarget.
Hook Punch (Gou Chong Chui): A punch delivered in a looping motion, usually targeting the opponent's jaw or temple.
Low Block (Hak Kiu): A defensive technique used to block or parry incoming low strikes.
High Block (Gau Kiu): A defensive technique used to block or parry incoming high strikes.
Sweeping Leg Takedown (Chen Tui): A technique

used to sweep the opponent's leg and bring them down to the ground.Reverse Punch (Fan Chong Chui): A punch executed with the rear hand, generating power from the rotation of the hips andtorso.

Butterfly Kick (Hudie Tui): A complex acrobatic kick involving a twisting motion of the body and amid-airrotation.

Iron Palm Strike (Tie Zhang Chui): A specialized strike developed through rigorous training to strengthen the palm for maximum impact. Tiger Claw Strike (Hu Zhua Chui): A strike resembling a claw using the fingers and palm, targeting soft tissue areas. Snake Hand Strike (She Shou Chui): A quick and precise strike executed with the fingers extended and the hand resembling a snake's head. Dragon Sweeps Its Tail (Long Xie Wei Bu): A sweeping motion performed with the leg, imitating the movement of a dragon's tail. Eagle Claw Grip (Ying Zhao Shou): A technique that involves using the fingers to grab and control an opponent's limbs or pressure points. Monkey Steals Peach (Hou Diao Tao): A quick grab or strike targeting the opponent's groin or sensitive areas, resembling a monkey's action. Drunken Fist (Zui Quan): A unique and deceptive style that mimics the movements and behavior of a drunken person, combining fluid strikes and unpredictablefootwork.

These techniques represent a variety of strikes, kicks, blocks, and grappling techniques found in Kung Fu. Remember that proper training, guidance, and practice are essential to mastering these techniques effectively.

1 Straight Punch (Jik Chong Chui):

A basic punch delivered straight from the shoulder with the knuckles as the striking point.
The Straight Punch, also known as Jik Chong Chui in Kung Fu, is a fundamental technique used in various martial arts styles, including Wing Chun, Shaolin, and Jeet Kune Do. It is a direct and powerful punch that aims to strike the opponent with maximum force. Here are the details of the Straight Punch technique:
The Straight Punch, also known as Jik Chong Chui in Kung Fu, is a fundamental technique used in various martial arts styles, including Wing Chun, Shaolin, and Jeet Kune Do. It is a direct and powerful punch that aims to strike the opponent with maximum force. Here are the details of the Straight Punch technique:

Stance: Begin in a solid and balanced stance, such as a front stance or a modified horse stance. Keep your feet shoulder-width apart, knees slightly bent, and body relaxed but ready.

Hand Position: Start with your fists guarding your chin, close to your face. The lead hand (the hand on the same side as your lead leg) should be positioned slightly forward, with the elbow bent at a 90-degree angle. The rear hand (on the opposite side) should be positioned closer to your chin, ready to deliver the punch.

Weight Transfer: Initiate the punch by shifting your weight from your back leg to your front leg. As you transfer your weight forward, rotate your hips and torso slightly to generate power.

Extension: Simultaneously extend your lead hand forward in a straight line, targeting the intended striking point. Keep your wrist straight and aligned with your forearm, and your knuckles should be the primary contact point.

Alignment: Ensure that your shoulder, elbow, wrist, and knuckles are in alignment as you extend your arm. This alignment optimizes the transfer of power and minimizes the risk of injury.

Recoil: After the punch lands or reaches its maximum extension, quickly retract your hand back to the starting position. This recoil movement should be snappy and controlled, allowing you to defend or deliver subsequent strikes.

Breathing: Coordinate your breath with the execution of the punch. Exhale sharply as you extend your arm, which helps to generate more power and maintain focus.

Focus Points: The Straight Punch can target various areas depending on the situation and style being practiced. Common targets include the solar plexus, chin, nose, or throat. However, it's essential to practice control and accuracy while training to avoid causing harm.

Speed and Power: With consistent practice, focus on improving the speed and power of your Straight Punch. Develop your ability to deliver fast and explosive strikes while maintaining proper technique and control.

Practice Drills: To refine your Straight Punch, practice shadowboxing, hitting focus mitts, or working with a training partner using controlled sparring drills. These drills allow you to develop accuracy, timing, and adaptability in real-time scenarios.

Remember, mastering the Straight Punch requires dedication, practice, and guidance from a qualified instructor. They can provide personalized feedback, correct any errors, and help you refine your technique for maximum effectiveness.

2 Palm Strike (Zhang Chui): A strike using the palm of the hand, often used for targeting sensitive areas like the nose or throat.

Certainly! Here's a detailed explanation of the Palm Strike technique, known as Zhang Chui in Kung Fu.

Stance: Start in a solid and balanced stance, such as a front stance or a modified horse stance. Keep your feet shoulder-width apart, knees slightly bent, and your body relaxed but ready.

Hand Position: Position your hands in a guarding position, with your palms facing inward and close to your chest. Your fingers should be slightly bent and ready to strike.

Weight Transfer: Transfer your weight from your back leg to your front leg as you initiate the strike. This weight transfer generates power and propels your strike forward.

Hand Movement: From the guarding position, rapidly extend your lead hand (the hand on the same side as your lead leg) forward in a straight line. Open your hand and turn it so that your palm faces outward, away from your body.

Striking Surface: The striking surface in a Palm

Strike is the fleshy part at the base of your palm, just below the thumb. This area is used to deliver the strike with maximum impact.

Arm Alignment: Maintain a straight line from your shoulder to your palm as you extend your arm. This alignment maximizes the transfer of power and ensures efficient delivery of force.

Contact and Follow-Through: As you extend your arm, drive your palm forward to make contact with the target. Aim to strike with the base of your palm, targeting areas like the nose, chin, throat, or solar plexus. Ensure that your strike is controlled and precise.

Recoil: After the strike, quickly retract your hand back to the guarding position. Maintain awareness and readiness for potential follow-up strikes or defensive actions.

Breathing: Coordinate your breath with the execution of the Palm Strike. Exhale sharply as you strike, which enhances power generation and focus.

Focus Points: The Palm Strike is effective in targeting vulnerable areas of the body. Common targets include the nose, chin, throat, sternum, or solar plexus. However, always exercise caution and control during training to avoid causing harm to your training partner.

Power Generation: Generating power in a Palm Strike primarily relies on body mechanics and weight transfer. Coordinate the movement of your hips, torso, and arm to generate power from the ground up.

Practice Drills: To refine your Palm Strike, practice on focus mitts or pads with a training partner. This allows you to develop accuracy, timing, and power while receiving feedback from your partner.

Application Variations: Kung Fu styles may have variations of the Palm Strike technique. For example, some styles incorporate simultaneous strikes with both hands or combine it with footwork for added effectiveness.

3 Front Kick (Chun Tui): A powerful kick executed by raising the knee and extending the leg straight forward.

The Front Kick, known as Chun Tui in Kung Fu, is a powerful kicking technique commonly used in martial arts. It involves raising the knee and extending the leg straight forward to strike the opponent or target. Here's a detailed breakdown of the Front Kick technique:

Stance: Begin in a balanced and stable stance, such as a front stance or a modified horse stance. Keep your feet shoulder-width apart, knees slightly bent, and your body relaxed but ready.

Chambering: Lift your knee of the kicking leg toward your chest, keeping it bent and close to your body. This position is known as the chambering position and prepares you for the kick.

Extension: From the chambering position, forcefully extend your leg forward in a straight line. Straighten your knee and deliver the kick using the ball of your foot or the top of your foot as the striking surface. Keep your toes pointed back and your ankle locked for optimal striking power and accuracy.

Hip Rotation: As you extend your leg,

simultaneously rotate your hip and torso in the direction of the kick. This rotation generates additional power and adds momentum to the kick.

Target Selection: The Front Kick can target various areas, depending on the situation and style being practiced. Common targets include the groin, abdomen, solar plexus, or chest. However, always exercise control and precision during training to avoid causing harm.

Recoil: After the kick lands or reaches its maximum extension, quickly retract your leg back to the chambering position. Maintain balance and readiness for further strikes or defensive actions.

Balance and Posture: Throughout the execution of the Front Kick, maintain a good sense of balance and posture. Keep your standing leg slightly bent and your upper body upright to enhance stability and control.

Breathing: Coordinate your breath with the execution of the kick. Exhale sharply as you extend your leg, which aids in generating power and maintaining focus.

Height Variation: Depending on the target or situation, you can vary the height of your Front Kick. It can be delivered low to strike the opponent's leg or mid to high levels to target the body or head. Practice adjusting the kick's trajectory and height to adapt to different scenarios.

Practice Drills: To improve your Front Kick, practice with a training partner using focus mitts or pads. This allows you to develop accuracy, timing, and power while receiving feedback from your   partner.

Flexibility and Strength: Regular stretching exercises and strength training can enhance the effectiveness and range of your Front Kick. Focus on developing flexibility in your hip flexors and leg muscles to achieve higher kicks and optimal performance.

Remember, mastering the Front Kick requires consistent practice, attention to detail, and guidance from a qualified instructor. They can provide personalized feedback, correct any errors, and help you refine your technique for maximum effectiveness.

4 Side Kick (Yao Tui): A kick delivered by extending the leg out to the side while maintaining   balance.
The Side Kick, known as Yao Tui in Kung Fu, is a dynamic kicking technique where the leg is extended out to the side while maintaining balance. It is a powerful and versatile kick used in various martial arts styles. Here's a detailed breakdown of the Side Kick technique.Stance: Begin in a balanced and stable stance, such as a front stance or a modified horse stance. Keep your feet shoulder-width apart, knees slightly bent, and your body relaxed but ready.

Chambering: Lift your knee of the kicking leg up and across your body, bending it at a 90-degree angle. This position is known as the chambering position and prepares you for the kick.

Extension: From the chambering position, forcefully extend your leg out to the side, away from your body. Straighten your knee and deliver the kick using the heel or the blade of your foot as the striking surface. Keep your toes pointed back and your ankle locked for optimal striking   power   and   accuracy.

Hip Rotation: As you extend your leg, simultaneously rotate your hip and torso in the direction of the kick. This rotation generates additional power and adds momentum to the kick. The rotation should be in the opposite direction of the kick.

Target Selection: The Side Kick can target various areas, depending on the situation and style being practiced. Common targets include the ribs, midsection, hip, or thigh of the opponent. However, always exercise control and precision during training to avoid causing harm.

Balance and Posture: Maintain a good sense of balance and posture throughout the execution of the Side Kick. Keep your standing leg slightly bent and your upper body upright to enhance stability and control.

Chambering Arm: As you chamber the kicking leg, the arm on the same side should extend diagonally across your body, providing balance and counterbalance to the kick.

Recoil: After the kick lands or reaches its maximum extension, quickly retract your leg back to the chambering position. Maintain balance and readiness for further strikes or defensive actions.

Breathing: Coordinate your breath with the execution of the kick. Exhale sharply as you extend your leg, which aids in generating power and maintaining focus.

Height Variation: The Side Kick can be executed at different heights, depending on the target or situation. Practice adjusting the kick's height to adapt to different scenarios, ranging from low to high levels.

Practice Drills: To improve your Side Kick, practice with a training partner using focus mitts or pads. This allows you to develop accuracy, timing, and power while receiving feedback from your partner.

Flexibility and Strength: Regular stretching exercises and strength training can enhance the effectiveness and range of your Side Kick. Focus on developing flexibility in your hips, hamstrings, and leg muscles to achieve higher kicks and optimal performance.

5 Roundhouse Kick (Waai Tui): A circular kick where the leg is swung around in a horizontal arc to strike the opponent.

The Roundhouse Kick, known as Waai Tui in Kung Fu, is a powerful and versatile kicking technique. It involves swinging the leg in a horizontal arc to strike the opponent. Here's a detailed breakdown of the Roundhouse Kick technique.

Stance: Begin in a balanced and stable stance, such as a front stance or a modified horse stance. Keep your feet shoulder-width apart, knees slightly bent, and your body relaxed but ready.

Chambering: Lift your knee of the kicking leg up towards your chest, bending it at a 90-degree angle. This chambering position prepares you for the   kick.

Arc and Rotation: From the chambering position, swing your leg in a horizontal arc, extending it out towards the target. As you swing, rotate your hips and pivot on the support leg, allowing your body to turn with the kick. The rotation generates power and adds momentum to the kick.

Striking Surface: The striking surface in a Roundhouse Kick can vary. It can be executed with the instep, ball of the foot, or the lower shin depending on the target and personal preference. Aim to strike with a firm and controlled impact.

Hip and Torso Rotation: As you swing your leg, engage your hip and torso rotation in the direction of the kick. This rotation enhances the power and speed of the kick and allows for proper alignment of the striking surface.

Target Selection: The Roundhouse Kick can target various areas, depending on the situation and style being practiced. Common targets include the midsection, ribs, thighs, or head. Ensure control and precision during training to avoid causing harm.

Chambering Arm: As you chamber the kicking leg, the arm on the same side should also be chambered. This helps with balance and counterbalance during the kick.

Guard and Balance: Keep your non-kicking hand up to protect your face and maintain a good sense of balance and posture throughout the execution of the Roundhouse Kick. Maintain a slightly bent standing leg and an upright upper body for stability.

Recoil: After the kick lands or reaches its maximum extension, quickly retract your leg back to the chambering position. Maintain balance and readiness for further strikes or defensive actions.

Breathing: Coordinate your breath with the execution of the kick. Exhale sharply as you extend your leg, which aids in generating power and maintaining focus.

Height Variation: The Roundhouse Kick can be executed at different heights, depending on the target or situation. Practice adjusting the kick's trajectory to adapt to different scenarios, ranging from low to mid to high levels.

Practice Drills: To improve your Roundhouse Kick, practice with a training partner using focus mitts or pads. This allows you to develop accuracy, timing, and power while receiving feedback from your partner.

Flexibility and Strength: Regular stretching exercises and strength training can enhance the effectiveness and range of your Roundhouse Kick. Focus on developing flexibility in your hip flexors, hamstrings, and leg muscles to achieve higher kicks and optimal performance.

6 Elbow Strike (Zhou Chui): A close-range strike using the elbow, typically directed at the opponent's vital areas.

The Elbow Strike, known as Zhou Chui in Kung Fu, is a close-range strike that utilizes the elbow as the striking point. It is a powerful technique commonly used in self-defense and close-quarters combat. Here's a detailed breakdown of the Elbow Strike technique:

Stance: Begin in a balanced and stable stance, such as a front stance or a modified horse stance. Keep your feet shoulder-width apart, knees slightly bent, and your body relaxed but ready.

Close the Gap: To execute an Elbow Strike effectively, close the distance between you and your opponent. Step in or use footwork to close the gap and bring yourself into range for the strike.

Target Selection: The Elbow Strike is typically directed at the opponent's vital areas. Common targets include the temple, jaw, nose, chin, solar plexus, ribs, or collarbone. Identify the vulnerable areas on your opponent and aim your strike accordingly.

Chambering: Chamber the elbow of your striking arm by bending it and positioning it close to your body. Keep your other hand up for guard and balance.

Extension: Extend your elbow forward forcefully, driving it towards the target. As you extend your elbow, generate power by rotating your hips and torso in the direction of the strike. This rotational force amplifies the impact of the strike.

Striking Surface: The striking surface in an Elbow Strike is the bony part of the elbow. Aim to strike with the tip or point of the elbow, which is the most effective and strongest part of the elbow.

Accuracy and Precision: Focus on delivering accurate and precise strikes. Aim to hit the target with the intended part of your elbow, concentrating on the specific area you are targeting.

Recoil: After the strike lands or reaches its maximum extension, quickly retract your elbow back to the chambering position. Maintain balance and readiness for further strikes or defensive actions.

Guard and Balance: Keep your non-striking hand up to protect your face and maintain a good sense of balance and posture throughout the execution of the Elbow Strike. Maintain a slightly bent standing leg and an upright upper body for stability.

Breathing: Coordinate your breath with the execution of the strike. Exhale sharply as you extend your elbow, which aids in generating power and maintaining focus.

Close-Quarters Training: Practice Elbow Strikes in close-quarters scenarios and drills. This helps develop the ability to strike effectively in confined spaces and simulate realistic combat situations.

Practice Drills: Train with a partner or focus mitts to practice and refine your Elbow Strikes. Focus on accuracy, speed, and generating power through proper body mechanics.

Strength and Conditioning: Strengthen your elbow joint and related muscles through conditioning exercises such as elbow push-ups and resistance training. This helps improve the effectiveness and endurance of your Elbow Strikes.

7 Knee Strike (Tui Chui): A strike using the knee, performed by raising the knee and driving it into the target.The Knee Strike, known as Tui Chui in Kung Fu, is a powerful strike that utilizes the knee as the striking point. It is a close-range technique that can be devastating when executed with proper technique and control. Here's a detailed breakdown of the Knee Strike technique:

Stance: Begin in a balanced and stable stance, such as a front stance or a modified horse stance. Keep your feet shoulder-width apart, knees slightly bent, and your body relaxed but ready.

Close the Gap: To perform a Knee Strike effectively, close the distance between you and your opponent. Step in or use footwork to bring yourself into range for the strike.

Target Selection: The Knee Strike can be directed at various targets, depending on the situation and style being practiced. Common targets include the groin, abdomen, thighs, or midsection of the opponent. Aim for vulnerable areas to maximize the effectiveness of your strike.

Chambering: Lift your knee of the striking leg towards your chest, bending it at a 90-degree angle. This chambering position prepares you for the strike.

Extension: Drive your knee forward forcefully, extending it towards the target. Simultaneously, generate power by rotating your hips and torso in the direction of the strike. This rotational force adds momentum and power to the Knee Strike.

Striking Surface: The striking surface in a Knee Strike is the lower part of your knee joint, below the patella (knee cap). Aim to strike with the bony part of your knee for maximum impact.

Accuracy and Precision: Focus on delivering accurate and precise strikes. Aim to hit the intended target with the center or lower part of your knee, concentrating on the specific area you are targeting.

Guard and Balance: Keep your non-striking hand up to protect your face and maintain a good sense of balance and posture throughout the execution of the Knee Strike. Ensure that your standing leg is slightly bent and your upper body remains upright for stability.

Recoil: After the strike lands or reaches its maximum extension, quickly retract your knee back to the chambering position. Maintain balance and readiness for further strikes or defensive actions.

Breathing: Coordinate your breath with the execution of the strike. Exhale sharply as you extend your knee, which aids in generating power and maintaining focus.

Close-Quarters Training: Practice Knee Strikes in close-quarters scenarios and drills. This helps develop the ability to strike effectively in confined spaces and simulate realistic combat situations.

Practice Drills: Train with a partner or focus mitts to practice and refine your Knee Strikes. Focus on accuracy, speed, and generating power through proper body mechanics.

Strength and Conditioning: Strengthen your leg muscles and improve knee joint stability through exercises such as squats, lunges, and leg presses. This helps enhance the power and stability of your Knee Strikes.

8 Hook Punch (Gou Chong Chui): A punch delivered in a looping motion, usually targeting the opponent's jaw or temple. The Hook Punch, known as Gou Chong Chui in Kung Fu, is a dynamic and powerful punch delivered in a looping motion. It is often used to target the opponent's jaw or temple. Here's a detailed breakdown of the Hook Punch technique.

Stance: Begin in a balanced and stable stance, such as a front stance or a modified horse stance. Keep your feet shoulder-width apart, knees slightly bent, and your body relaxed but ready.

Hand Position: Position your lead hand (the hand on the same side as your lead leg) slightly in front of your face, with the elbow bent at a 90-degree angle. Keep your rear hand (on the opposite side) close to your chin to protect your face.

Weight Transfer: Initiate the punch by shifting your weight from your back leg to your front leg. As you transfer your weight forward, rotate your hips and torso slightly to generate power.

Looping Motion: As you rotate your hips and torso, extend your lead arm in a looping motion.

Imagine drawing a semi-circular arc with your fist, aiming to strike the opponent's jaw or temple. The punch should travel in a circular or hooking trajectory.

Striking Surface: The striking surface in a Hook Punch is the first two knuckles of your closed fist. These knuckles are aligned with your index and middle fingers. Aim to strike with the side of your fist, making contact with the intended target.

Alignment: Ensure that your shoulder, elbow, wrist, and knuckles are in alignment as you extend your arm. This alignment optimizes the transfer of power and minimizes the risk of injury.

Recoil: After the punch lands or reaches its maximum extension, quickly retract your arm back to the starting position. Maintain balance and readiness for further strikes or defensive actions.

Breathing: Coordinate your breath with the execution of the punch. Exhale sharply as you extend your arm, which helps generate more power and maintain focus.

Target Selection: The Hook Punch primarily targets the opponent's jaw or temple, aiming to disrupt their balance and potentially cause injury. Practice control and accuracy during training to avoid causing harm to your training partner.

Guard and Balance: Keep your non-striking hand up to protect your face and maintain a good sense of balance and posture throughout the execution of the Hook Punch. Ensure that your standing leg is slightly bent and your upper body remains upright for stability.

Practice Drills: Train with a partner or focus mitts to practice and refine your Hook Punch. Focus on accuracy, timing, and generating power through proper body mechanics.

Speed and Power: With consistent practice, focus on improving the speed and power of your Hook Punch. Develop the ability to deliver fast and explosive strikes while maintaining proper technique and control.

9 Low Block (Hak Kiu): A defensive technique used to block or parry incoming low strikes. The Low Block, known as Hak Kiu in Kung Fu, is a defensive technique used to block or parry incoming low strikes. It is designed to protect your lower body, particularly the legs and lower torso, from kicks, sweeps, or strikes aimed at those areas. Here's a detailed breakdown of the Low Block technique:

Stance: Begin in a balanced and stable stance, such as a front stance or a modified horse stance. Keep your feet shoulder-width apart, knees slightly bent, and your body relaxed but ready.

Hand Position: Position your arms in a guarding position, with your fists closed and your elbows bent at approximately 90 degrees. Place your hands in front of your lower body, just below the waist, with your palms facing upward.

Movement: When executing the Low Block, initiate the movement from your elbows and forearms. Simultaneously bring your forearms downward and inward in a diagonal motion across your body. The blocking motion should be firm, controlled, and executed with speed.

Blocking Surface: The blocking surface in a Low Block is the outer or upper portion of your forearm. Position it to intercept and deflect incoming strikes or kicks aimed at your lower body.

Angle and Position: Position your blocking forearm at a diagonal angle to effectively intercept the incoming strike. The exact angle and position will depend on the direction and height of the attack. Practice adapting the angle and position to various scenarios.

Timing: Time your Low Block to meet the incoming strike at the optimal moment. Execute the block just before the strike connects to effectively intercept and redirect the attack.

Recoil: After the block, quickly return your forearm to the starting position. Maintain readiness for further defensive actions or counterattacks.

Balance and Posture: Maintain a good sense of balance and posture throughout the execution of the Low Block. Keep your knees slightly bent and your upper body upright to enhance stability and control.

Breathing: Coordinate your breath with the execution of the block. Exhale naturally during the block, which aids in focus and relaxation.

Target Area: The Low Block is primarily used to defend against strikes aimed at your lower body, such as low kicks or sweeps. Practice control and accuracy to intercept the attack effectively.

Practice Drills: Train with a partner or focus mitts to practice and refine your Low Block technique. Focus on accuracy, timing, and developing the ability to react quickly to incoming strikes.

Fluid Transitions: Combine the Low Block with other defensive and offensive techniques to create fluid transitions. Work on smoothly transitioning from blocking to counterattacking or follow-up defensive movements.

10 High Block (Gau Kiu): A defensive technique used to block or parry incoming high strikes. The High Block, known as Gau Kiu in Kung Fu, is a defensive technique used to block or parry incoming high strikes. It is designed to protect your upper body, particularly your head, neck, and upper torso, from strikes such as punches or strikes aimed at those areas. Here's a detailed breakdown of the High Block technique: The High Block, known as Gau Kiu in Kung Fu, is a defensive technique used to block or parry incoming high strikes. It is designed to protect your upper body, particularly your head, neck, and upper torso, from strikes such as punches or strikes aimed at those areas. Here's a detailed breakdown of the High Block technique:

Stance: Begin in a balanced and stable stance, such as a front stance or a modified horse stance. Keep your feet shoulder-width apart, knees slightly bent, and your body relaxed but ready.

Hand Position: Position your arms in a guarding position, with your fists closed and your elbows bent at approximately 90 degrees. Place your hands in front of your face, with your palms facing inward and your fists positioned at the sides of your forehead.

Movement: When executing the High Block,

initiate the movement from your elbows and forearms. Simultaneously bring your forearms upward and outward in a diagonal motion across your body. The blocking motion should be firm, controlled, and executed with speed.

Blocking Surface: The blocking surface in a High Block is the outer or upper portion of your forearm. Position it to intercept and deflect incoming strikes or punches aimed at your upper body.

Angle and Position: Position your blocking forearm at a diagonal angle to effectively intercept the incoming strike. The exact angle and position will depend on the direction and height of the attack. Practice adapting the angle and position to various scenarios.

Timing: Time your High Block to meet the incoming strike at the optimal moment. Execute the block just before the strike connects to effectively intercept and redirect the attack.

Recoil: After the block, quickly return your forearm to the starting position. Maintain readiness for further defensive actions or counterattacks.

Balance and Posture: Maintain a good sense of balance and posture throughout the execution of the High Block. Keep your knees slightly bent and your upper body upright to enhance stability and control.

Breathing: Coordinate your breath with the execution of the block. Exhale naturally during the block, which aids in focus and relaxation.

Target Area: The High Block is primarily used to defend against strikes aimed at your upper body, such as punches or strikes targeting your head, neck, or chest. Practice control and accuracy to intercept the attack effectively.

Practice Drills: Train with a partner or focus mitts to practice and refine your High Block technique. Focus on accuracy, timing, and developing the ability to react quickly to incoming strikes.

Fluid Transitions: Combine the High Block with other defensive and offensive techniques to create fluid transitions. Work on smoothly transitioning from blocking to counterattacking or follow-up defensive movements.

11 Sweeping Leg Takedown (Chen Tui): A technique used to sweep the opponent's leg and bring them down to the ground.

The Sweeping Leg Takedown, known as Chen Tui in Kung Fu, is a technique used to sweep the opponent's leg and bring them down to the ground. It is an effective method of off-balancing an opponent and gaining control in close-quarters combat. Here's a detailed breakdown of the Sweeping Leg Takedown technique:

Stance: Begin in a balanced and stable stance, such as a front stance or a modified horse stance. Keep your feet shoulder-width apart, knees slightly bent, and your body relaxed but ready.

Gripping and Control: Before attempting the sweep, establish a grip or control on the opponent's upper body or arms. This grip helps you maintain control and disrupt their balance during the takedown.

Timing and Distraction: Create a momentary distraction or off-balance the opponent to make them vulnerable to the sweep. This can be done through feints, strikes, or redirecting their energy.

Leg Placement: Position your sweeping leg on the same side as your gripping hand. It should be positioned outside the opponent's leg, allowing you to effectively sweep their leg from the outside.

Sweep Motion: With a quick and fluid motion, swing your sweeping leg in a semicircular or hooking motion, aiming to strike the back of the opponent's supporting leg. Maintain control of the upper body or arms to further disrupt their balance.

Power Generation: Generate power for the sweep by utilizing your hip and torso rotation. Coordinate the movement of your hips and upper body with the swing of your sweeping leg to maximize the force of the takedown.

Follow-Through: As your sweeping leg makes contact with the opponent's leg, continue the sweeping motion by driving through their leg, causing them to lose balance and fall to the ground. Be sure to maintain your own balance and control throughout the motion.

Maintain Control: Once the opponent is brought

down to the ground, ensure that you maintain control of their upper body or arms to prevent them from recovering quickly or countering.

Protect Yourself: As you execute the takedown, be aware of the potential for the opponent to counter or attempt to grab onto you. Maintain good posture and be prepared to defend or transition to a more advantageous position.

Practice Drills: Train with a partner to practice and refine your Sweeping Leg Takedown technique. Start with slow and controlled movements before progressing to more dynamic and realistic scenarios.

Timing and Footwork: Develop proper timing and footwork to execute the sweep effectively. Practice anticipating the opponent's movement and utilizing footwork to position yourself for a successful takedown.

Safety and Control: When training the Sweeping Leg Takedown, prioritize safety and control. Gradually increase the speed and intensity of the takedown as you gain proficiency and confidence.

12 Reverse Punch (Fan Chong Chui): A punch executed with the rear hand, generating power from the rotation of the hips and torso.

The Reverse Punch, known as Fan Chong Chui in Kung Fu, is a powerful punch executed with the rear hand. It generates power from the rotation of the hips and torso. This technique is commonly used in martial arts to deliver strong and accurate strikes. Here's a detailed breakdown of the Reverse Punch technique:

Stance: Begin in a balanced and stable stance, such as a front stance or a modified horse stance. Keep your feet shoulder-width apart, knees slightly bent, and your body relaxed but ready.

Hand Position: Position your lead hand (the hand on the same side as your lead leg) slightly in front of your face, with the elbow bent at approximately 90 degrees. Keep your rear hand (on the opposite side) close to your chin to protect your face.

Weight Transfer: Initiate the punch by shifting your weight from your front leg to your back leg. As you transfer your weight backward, rotate your hips and torso in the direction of the punch.

This hip and torso rotation generates power for the strike.

Chambering: As you rotate your hips and torso, simultaneously pull your rear hand back toward your hip. This position is the chambering position and prepares your hand for the punch.

Extension: From the chambering position, extend your rear hand forward in a straight line, rotating your shoulder, arm, and fist as you drive the punch. As you extend, rotate your palm to face downward, aligning your knuckles for impact.

Striking Surface: The striking surface in a Reverse Punch is the first two knuckles of your closed fist. These knuckles are aligned with your index and middle fingers. Aim to strike with the first two knuckles for optimal power and alignment.

Arm Alignment: Ensure that your shoulder, elbow, wrist, and knuckles are in alignment as you extend your arm. This alignment optimizes power transfer and reduces the risk of injury.

Recoil: After the punch lands or reaches its

maximum extension, quickly retract your hand back to the chambering position. Maintain balance and readiness for further strikes or defensive actions.

Breathing: Coordinate your breath with the execution of the punch. Exhale sharply as you extend your arm, which aids in generating power and maintaining focus.

Accuracy and Precision: Focus on delivering accurate and precise strikes. Aim to hit the target with the first two knuckles of your fist, concentrating on specific areas such as the jaw, temple, or solar plexus.

Guard and Balance: Keep your non-punching hand up to protect your face and maintain a good sense of balance and posture throughout the execution of the Reverse Punch. Ensure that your standing leg is slightly bent, and your upper body remains upright for stability.

Practice Drills: Train with a partner or focus mitts to practice and refine your Reverse Punch technique. Focus on accuracy, timing, and generating power through proper body mechanics.

Speed and Power: With consistent practice, focus on improving the speed and power of your Reverse Punch. Develop the ability to deliver fast and explosive strikes while maintaining proper technique and control.

13 Spinning Back Kick (Diu Tui): A powerful kick performed by spinning the body and striking the opponent with the heel of the foot.

The Spinning Back Kick, known as Diu Tui in Kung Fu, is a powerful and dynamic kick performed by spinning the body and striking the opponent with the heel of the foot. It is an effective technique used in various martial arts styles for both offensive and defensive purposes. Here's a detailed breakdown of the Spinning Back Kick technique:

Stance: Begin in a balanced and stable stance, such as a front stance or a modified horse stance. Keep your feet shoulder-width apart, knees slightly bent, and your body relaxed but ready.

Set-Up: Position yourself so that your opponent is within striking range. Maintain focus on your target while keeping your guard up to protect yourself.

Chambering: As you prepare for the Spinning Back Kick, rotate your body in the direction opposite to the kick. Lift your knee of the kicking leg towards your chest, bending it at a 90-degree angle. This chambering position prepares you for

thekick.
Rotation: Initiate the spin by pivoting on the ball of your standing foot. Rotate your body in the direction opposite to the kick, using the power generated from your hips and torso to generate momentum.

Kick Extension: As your body rotates, forcefully extend your kicking leg out in a straight line, striking the opponent with the heel of your foot. Keep your toes pulled back and your ankle locked for optimal striking power and accuracy.

Striking Surface: The striking surface in a Spinning Back Kick is the heel of your foot. Aim to strike the opponent with the back of your heel, focusing on vulnerable areas such as the midsection, ribs, or head.

Hip and Torso Rotation: Coordinate the rotation of your hips and torso with the kick extension. This rotation generates additional power and adds momentum to the kick, increasing its effectiveness.

Accuracy and Precision: Focus on delivering accurate and precise strikes. Visualize your target and aim to hit with the heel of your foot, concentrating on the specific area you are targeting.

Recoil and Recovery: After the kick lands or reaches its maximum extension, quickly bring your kicking leg back to the chambering position and regain your balance. Maintain readiness for further strikes or defensive actions.

Guard and Balance: Keep your non-kicking hand up to protect your face and maintain a good sense of balance and posture throughout the execution of the Spinning Back Kick. Keep your standing leg slightly bent and your upper body upright for stability.

Breathing: Coordinate your breath with the execution of the kick. Exhale sharply as you extend your leg, which aids in generating power and maintaining focus.

Practice Drills: Train with a partner or focus mitts to practice and refine your Spinning Back Kick technique. Focus on accuracy, timing, and generating power through proper body mechanics.

Flexibility and Core Strength: Develop flexibility in your hip flexors and leg muscles through regular stretching exercises. Additionally, focus on core strength training to enhance the rotational power of your kick.

14 Tiger Claw Strike (Hu Zhua Chui): A strike resembling a claw using the fingers and palm, targeting soft tissue areas.

The Tiger Claw Strike, known as Hu Zhua Chui in Kung Fu, is a striking technique that resembles a claw using the fingers and palm. It is an aggressive and versatile strike often used to target soft tissue areas of the opponent's body. Here's a detailed breakdown of the Tiger Claw Strike technique:

Hand Position: Start by forming a claw-like hand shape, with your fingers slightly bent and your fingertips pointing towards the target. Keep your thumb slightly tucked in for support and stability.

Grip and Alignment: Ensure that your fingers are aligned and slightly spread apart, resembling the extended claws of a tiger. The fingertips and nails should be the primary striking points.

Target Selection: The Tiger Claw Strike is designed to target soft tissue areas of the opponent's body. Common targets include the face, eyes, throat, neck, groin, or any vulnerable area within striking range.

Striking Motion: Execute the strike by extending your arm with a quick and controlled motion. Focus on extending your fingers and driving the striking surface (fingertips and palm) towards the   target.

Raking or Grabbing Motion: The Tiger Claw Strike can be performed as a raking motion, where the fingers scrape or rake across the target, causing pain and discomfort. Alternatively, it can be used as a grabbing or clawing motion, where the fingers dig into the target to inflict damage and control the opponent.

Follow-Through: After making contact with the target, retract your hand quickly and maintain control of the situation. Be prepared to follow up with additional strikes or defensive actions.

Accuracy and Precision: Focus on delivering accurate strikes. Aim to hit the intended target with the fingertips or palm of your Tiger Claw Strike, concentrating on specific areas for maximum   effect.

Timing and Distance: Develop proper timing and

judgment of distance to execute the Tiger Claw Strike effectively. Practice anticipating the opponent's movements and adjust your strike accordingly.

Guard and Balance: Keep your non-striking hand up to protect your face and maintain a good sense of balance and posture throughout the execution of the strike. Stay alert and ready to defend against any counterattacks.

Breathing: Coordinate your breath with the execution of the strike. Exhale naturally as you strike, which aids in generating power and maintaining focus.

Practice Drills: Train with a partner or practice on target pads to refine your Tiger Claw Strike technique. Focus on accuracy, timing, and generating power through proper body mechanics.

Control and Safety: When practicing the Tiger Claw Strike, exercise control and ensure safety. Gradually increase the intensity of your strikes as you become more comfortable and skilled.

15 Snake Hand Strike (She Shou Chui): A quick and precise strike executed with the fingers extended and the hand resembling a snake's head.

The Snake Hand Strike, known as She Shou Chui in Kung Fu, is a quick and precise strike executed with the fingers extended and the hand resembling a snake's head. It is a deceptive and versatile technique used to target vulnerable areas of the opponent's body. Here's a detailed breakdown of the Snake Hand Strike technique:

Hand Position: Start by extending your fingers, keeping them close together and slightly bent. The hand should resemble the shape of a snake's head, with the fingertips forming the striking point.

Target Selection: The Snake Hand Strike is typically used to target vital areas of the opponent's body, such as the eyes, throat, solar plexus, or nerve clusters. Aim for soft and sensitive areas for maximum effectiveness.

Striking Motion: Execute the strike by extending your arm in a quick and controlled manner. Focus on driving the fingertips forward, aiming to penetrate or strike the target with precision.

Precision and Accuracy: Pay attention to precision and accuracy in your strikes. Aim to hit the intended target with the fingertips of your Snake Hand Strike, focusing on specific areas to maximize the impact.

Speed and Deception: Emphasize speed and deception in your Snake Hand Strikes. Employ quick and unexpected movements to surprise your opponent and make your strikes harder to anticipate or defend against.

Recoil and Readiness: After making contact with the target, quickly retract your hand and return to a ready position. Maintain your focus and be prepared for further strikes or defensive actions.

Timing and Distance: Develop a sense of timing and judgment of distance to execute the Snake Hand Strike effectively. Practice your strikes at various distances to gauge the appropriate reach and timing required.

Guard and Balance: Keep your non-striking hand up to protect your face and maintain a good sense of balance and posture throughout the execution of the strike. Stay alert and ready to defend against any counterattacks.

Breathing: Coordinate your breath with the execution of the strike. Exhale naturally as you strike, which aids in generating power and maintaining focus.

Practice Drills: Train with a partner or practice on target pads to refine your Snake Hand Strike technique. Focus on accuracy, timing, and generating power through proper body mechanics.

Control and Safety: When practicing the Snake Hand Strike, exercise control and ensure safety. Gradually increase the intensity of your strikes as you become more comfortable and skilled.

Awareness and Adaptability: Develop awareness of the opponent's movements and adapt your Snake Hand Strikes accordingly. Observe openings and vulnerabilities in their defense to maximize the effectiveness of your strikes.

16 Wing Chun Chain Punch (Yong Chun Sao Chui): A rapid succession of straight punches delivered from a close fighting position.

The Wing Chun Chain Punch, known as Yong Chun Sao Chui in Kung Fu, is a rapid succession of straight punches delivered from a close fighting position. It is a hallmark technique of Wing Chun Kung Fu, known for its speed, precision, and relentless attack. Here's a detailed breakdown of the Wing Chun Chain Punch technique:

Stance: Begin in a balanced and stable Wing Chun stance, such as the Yee Jee Kim Yeung Ma or the Bil Jee stance. Keep your feet shoulder-width apart, knees slightly bent, and your body relaxed but ready.

Centerline Focus: Wing Chun emphasizes the concept of the centerline, which is an imaginary line running down the middle of your body. Keep your punches directed along this line to maximize efficiency and accuracy.

Guard Position: Place your lead hand in a high guard position, positioned near your face and along the centerline. Keep your rear hand close to your chest to protect your body.

Rapid Succession: Execute a rapid series of straight punches with both hands, alternating between the lead and rear hand. Each punch should be delivered with speed and precision, allowing for minimal telegraphing and maximum efficiency.

Hand Positioning: As one hand punches forward, the other hand retracts to the guard position. The punches should originate from the shoulder, extending the arm along the centerline. Keep your punches compact and straight, minimizing unnecessary movement.

Hip and Torso Rotation: Coordinate the rotation of your hips and torso with each punch. Generate power by driving the rotation from your core, transferring it through your shoulders and into your arms. This rotational force enhances the impact and speed of your punches.

Breathing: Coordinate your breath with the execution of the chain punches. Exhale sharply with each punch, which aids in generating power and maintaining focus.

Accuracy and Precision: Focus on delivering accurate and precise punches. Aim to hit the intended target with the first two knuckles of your closed fist, concentrating on specific areas such as the solar plexus, jaw, or chin.

Continuous Flow: Maintain a continuous flow of punches, minimizing any pauses between strikes. This relentless attack puts pressure on your opponent, disrupts their rhythm, and creates opportunities for further follow-up techniques.

Guard and Defense: Maintain a solid guard position with your non-punching hand, protecting your face and body. Maintain awareness of potential counterattacks and be ready to defend or redirect the opponent's strikes.

Core Strength and Conditioning: Develop core strength through exercises such as planks, sit-ups, and rotational exercises. A strong core enhances stability, power, and endurance for executing the Wing Chun Chain Punch.

Practice Drills: Train with a partner or focus mitts to practice and refine your Wing Chun

Chain Punch technique. Focus on maintaining speed, accuracy, and fluidity in your punches while maintaining proper form and control.

Remember, mastering the Wing Chun Chain Punch requires consistent practice, attention to detail, and guidance from a qualified instructor. They can provide personalized feedback, correct any errors in technique, and help you refine your punching skills for maximum effectiveness.

17 Butterfly Kick (Hudie Tui): A complex acrobatic kick involving a twisting motion of the body and a mid-air rotation.

The Butterfly Kick, known as Hudie Tui in Kung Fu, is a complex acrobatic kick that involves a twisting motion of the body and a mid-air rotation. It is a visually impressive technique that showcases agility, coordination, and athleticism. Here's a detailed breakdown of the Butterfly Kick technique:

Stance: Begin in a balanced and stable stance, such as a modified horse stance or a slight crouch. Keep your feet shoulder-width apart, knees slightly bent, and your body relaxed but ready.

Set-Up and Timing: Assess the distance and timing required for the Butterfly Kick. This kick is typically performed as a counterattack or as part of a combination, so be aware of the opponent's movements and create an opening to execute the kick.

Jump: Initiate the Butterfly Kick by jumping into the air using both legs. Push off from the ground with power and explosiveness to gain height and distance.

Body Positioning: As you jump, tuck your knees towards your chest and bring your feet close together, resembling a butterfly's wings. This position allows for easier rotation and enhances control during the kick.

Twisting Motion: During the mid-air phase of the kick, initiate a twisting motion of the body. Rotate your hips, torso, and shoulders in the direction opposite to your jump, creating the spin for the Butterfly Kick.

Kick Extension: As your body rotates in the air, extend one leg outward and perform a kicking motion. The extended leg should be straight and parallel to the ground, showcasing control and precision.

Kicking Surface: The striking surface in a Butterfly Kick is typically the inside edge of your foot, near the arch. However, variations can also involve striking with the ball of the foot or even the heel, depending on personal preference and style.

Spotting: Maintain focus and spot your landing

spot as you rotate in the air. This helps maintain control and balance throughout the kick, as well as ensures a safe landing.

Landing: As you complete the rotation and the kick reaches its maximum extension, prepare for a smooth and controlled landing. Extend your legs to absorb the impact and maintain balance upon touchdown.

Flexibility and Conditioning: Develop flexibility in your hips, legs, and core through regular stretching exercises. Strengthen your lower body and core muscles to enhance stability and control during the Butterfly Kick.

Safety and Progression: Practice the Butterfly Kick in a controlled and safe environment, ensuring that you have the necessary strength, flexibility, and skill level to perform the technique safely. Progress gradually, starting with basic variations and advancing to more complex forms as you gain proficiency.

Practice Drills: Train with a qualified instructor or experienced partner who can provide guidance and feedback. Use crash mats or other padded surfaces during the initial stages of learning to ensure safety and build confidence.

Remember, mastering the Butterfly Kick requires extensive practice, dedication, and guidance from a qualified instructor. Proper progressions and safety precautions should be followed to prevent injury and ensure steady improvement.

18 Iron Palm Strike (Tie Zhang Chui): A specialized strike developed through rigorous training to strengthen the palm for maximum impact.

The Iron Palm Strike, known as Tie Zhang Chui in Kung Fu, is a specialized strike developed through rigorous training to strengthen the palm for maximum impact. It is a powerful technique that focuses on conditioning the palm, increasing striking power, and delivering devastating blows. Here's a detailed breakdown of the Iron Palm Strike technique:

Preparation: Start by preparing your body for the training required to develop the Iron Palm Strike. This typically involves conditioning exercises to strengthen the hand, wrist, and forearm, as well as building overall physical fitness.

Hand Conditioning: Begin with basic hand conditioning exercises to toughen the skin and strengthen the palm. This may include striking a sandbag or a conditioning board, gradually increasing the intensity over time. Apply herbal liniments or dit da jow to promote healing and resilience.

Bone Conditioning: Incorporate bone conditioning techniques to strengthen the bones in your hand and make them more resistant to impact. This can involve striking various surfaces, such as iron bars or bean bags filled with pebbles, with controlled force and gradually increasing intensity.

Technique Training: Focus on proper technique while performing the Iron Palm Strike. Keep your hand relaxed, but firm, with the fingers slightly bent and the palm slightly cupped. The striking surface is primarily the heel of the palm, near the base of the fingers.

Body Alignment: Align your body properly to generate maximum power in the strike. Coordinate the movement of your hips, torso, and arm to transfer power from your lower body through the palm strike.

Breath Control: Coordinate your breath with the execution of the strike. Exhale sharply as you deliver the Iron Palm Strike, which aids in generating power and maintaining focus.

Target Selection: The Iron Palm Strike can target various areas, such as the torso, ribs, or head.

Practice control and accuracy to strike with the proper amount of force and precision.

Gradual Progression: Begin with lighter strikes and gradually increase the intensity and force as your hand conditioning progresses. Avoid rushing the process to prevent injuries and promote proper development.

Recovery and Healing: Allow adequate time for rest and recovery between training sessions to avoid overexertion and promote healing. Follow proper hand care techniques, such as applying herbal remedies and practicing hand exercises, to maintain the health and resilience of your palm.

Regular Practice: Consistency is key to developing the Iron Palm Strike. Practice regularly, dedicating specific training sessions to focus on the technique and conditioning of your palm.

Safety Precautions: Pay attention to safety precautions during training. Use appropriate protective gear, such as hand wraps or gloves, to minimize the risk of injury. Listen to your body and consult with a qualified instructor if you experience any pain or discomfort.

Seek Guidance: It is highly recommended to seek guidance from a qualified instructor experienced in Iron Palm training. They can provide personalized training programs, correct any errors in technique, and ensure your training progresses safely and effectively.

19 Dragon Sweeps Its Tail (Long Xie Wei Bu): A sweeping motion performed with the leg, imitating the movement of a dragon's tail.

The Dragon Sweeps Its Tail, known as Long Xie Wei Bu in Kung Fu, is a sweeping motion performed with the leg, imitating the movement of a dragon's tail. It is a dynamic and fluid technique used to off-balance opponents and create openings for further attacks. Here's a detailed breakdown of the Dragon Sweeps Its Tail technique:

Stance: Begin in a balanced and stable stance, such as a front stance or a modified horse stance. Keep your feet shoulder-width apart, knees slightly bent, and your body relaxed but ready.

Set-Up and Timing: Assess the distance and timing required for the Dragon Sweeps Its Tail technique. Create an opening or an opportunity to execute the sweep by manipulating the opponent's balance or exploiting their movement.

Chambering: As you prepare for the sweep, lift your sweeping leg and bend your knee, bringing your foot close to your buttocks. This chambering position sets up the motion and prepares your leg for the sweeping action.

Sweeping Motion: Initiate the sweeping motion by extending your leg outward and slightly downward in a controlled and fluid movement. Imagine the motion of a dragon's tail as it sweeps gracefully through the air.

Leg Positioning: Position your sweeping leg in a diagonal line across the opponent's lower body. Aim to make contact with the lower legs, ankles, or feet to disrupt their balance and stability.

Foot Position: The foot of your sweeping leg can be positioned with the toes pointing upward or downward, depending on the target and desired effect. Experiment with different angles to find the most effective position for the sweep.

Balance and Control: Maintain a good sense of balance and control throughout the sweeping motion. Keep your supporting leg stable and maintain proper posture to enhance stability and prevent yourself from being off-balanced.

Power Generation: Generate power for the sweep by utilizing the rotational movement of your hip and torso. Coordinate the movement of your hip and upper body with the extension of your leg to maximize the force and effectiveness of the sweep.

Timing and Distance: Develop a sense of timing and judgment of distance to execute the Dragon Sweeps Its Tail effectively. Practice anticipating the opponent's movements and adjusting your sweep accordingly.

Follow-Through: After the sweep, quickly retract your leg and regain your balance. Be prepared to follow up with additional strikes, kicks, or defensive actions as necessary.

Practice Drills: Train with a partner to practice and refine your Dragon Sweeps Its Tail technique. Focus on accuracy, timing, and developing the ability to react quickly to the opponent's movements.

Fluid Transitions: Combine the Dragon Sweeps Its Tail with other techniques to create fluid transitions. Practice smoothly transitioning from the sweep to other offensive or defensive movements, enhancing your overall fighting capability.

20 Eagle Claw Grip (Ying Zhao Shou): A technique that involves using the fingers to grab and control an opponent's limbs or pressure points.

The Eagle Claw Grip, known as Ying Zhao Shou in Kung Fu, is a technique that involves using the fingers to grab and control an opponent's limbs or pressure points. It is a versatile and precise technique that allows for joint manipulation, control, and application of pressure to vulnerable areas. Here's a detailed breakdown of the Eagle Claw Grip technique:

Hand Position: Begin by forming an Eagle Claw hand shape, with your fingers slightly bent and spread apart. The fingertips should resemble the claws of an eagle, ready to grasp and control the opponent.

Target Selection: The Eagle Claw Grip can be used to grab and control various areas of the opponent's body, such as their limbs, joints, or pressure points. Focus on vulnerable areas that can be targeted for manipulation or application of pressure.

Finger Control: Utilize the strength and dexterity of your fingers to grasp and secure the opponent's body. Aim to use all the fingers, including the thumb, to create a firm and secure grip.

Grabbing and Controlling Limbs: Use the Eagle Claw Grip to grab and control the opponent's limbs, such as their wrist, forearm, or biceps. Apply pressure or manipulation to restrict their movement and neutralize their attacks.

Joint Manipulation: Employ the Eagle Claw Grip to manipulate and control the joints of the opponent's body, such as their fingers, wrist, elbow, or shoulder. Apply twisting, pulling, or pushing motions to disrupt their balance and create opportunities for further techniques.

Pressure Point Activation: Utilize the Eagle Claw Grip to target and apply pressure to specific pressure points on the opponent's body. Apply firm but controlled pressure to sensitive areas to induce pain, discomfort, or temporary paralysis.

Sensitivity and Timing: Develop sensitivity and timing in applying the Eagle Claw Grip. Practice reading and adapting to the opponent's movements and responses, adjusting the grip and pressure accordingly.

Flow and Transitions: Combine the Eagle Claw Grip with other techniques to create fluid transitions. Practice smoothly transitioning from the grip to strikes, joint locks, or throws, enhancing your overall fighting ability.

Precision and Control: Focus on delivering precise and controlled grabs and manipulations. Avoid excessive force or unnecessary movements that may compromise your control or limit your options.

Practice Drills: Train with a partner to practice and refine your Eagle Claw Grip technique. Focus on accuracy, timing, and developing the ability to apply the grip in various scenarios and positions.

Safety and Control: When training the Eagle Claw Grip, prioritize safety and control. Practice gradually increasing the intensity and pressure to avoid injury and ensure proper development of the technique.

Seek Guidance: It is highly recommended to seek guidance from a qualified instructor experienced in Eagle Claw techniques. They can provide personalized training programs, correct any errors in technique, and ensure your training progresses safely and effectively.

www.ingramcontent.com/pod-product-compliance
Lightning Source LLC
Chambersburg PA
CBHW071611270726
48661CB00019B/2246